INTRODUCTION

Welcome to my world, fighting cancer. Shocking as it may be to hear those words, "You have cancer," it does take a while to get the mind around it. However, I'm telling you what I did to deal dealing with it. None of these statements have been validated or confirmed by the FDA. So please understand, everything said here is based on my opinions and my experience. I am not a doctor, so please do not consider this medical advice. Nothing I say to you may be approved by your specialist. If you are in treatment with lots of medicines, for example, like they gave to some poor unlucky fellow I know who has prostate cancer, I don't know what to tell you except, go slow. What the medical profession will not acknowledge is that supplements can help anyone or anybody.   I'm breathing heavily on 70 years of age. I've only heard of one doctor out of 50 who got cancer and did CRS (chemo, radiation, surgery). He did not live very long. So what are doctors doing to help themselves? Why does it appear to be a secret? We'll never know.

But let's start out with the basics. Medications are designed to alleviate symptoms by masking symptoms. If you have pain, you take a pain pill. It's great if you can take medications. However, in my world of taking medications, for every action there is an equal and opposite reaction. I take a third of a Children's Tylenol, and I have major GI distress. I take Zofran, and I'm so constipated my eyes turn black. So trust me when I tell you that what I'm doing for my cancers, pleural, does not make me sick in the least or throw me into a deep medicated state.

My cancer has been in my body for years just waiting to strike. It laid dormant in my left eye for over 30 years. Then suddenly when I requested a physical due to heart pounding in my ears, that's when tests were conducted and I was told, you have metastatic melanoma not only in your eye, but in your lung. It's metastatic, and you have six to eight weeks to live.

Please keep in mind. You have trillions of cells in your body. Where do you start? I was so nauseated that the smell of food cooking was disgusting. I did something good for me. Three weeks later, odors were not an issue.

I will tell you now and again and again. Whenever you take anything new whether, it's an ibuprofen, a Tylenol, pain pill, anything new that you ingest, take it slow and easy. It could cause a sickly reaction. Prescription drugs can cause such a nasty reaction in your body it could kill you, but that doesn't happen with alternative therapies. You might get a rash, feel a little sick.

However, I have heard of death by prescription drugs. Have you ever seen what an adverse or allergic reaction does to a body? I had a case of tongue rolling for 12 hours with a medicine I took years ago for stomach problems. It was nasty. When I talked to the FDA, they said, reported issues have to be more than a certain percentage to get it off the market. How many people never call? How many people have to die before a drug is pulled?

My best free advice to you is, do NOT be overzealous in starting something new. Start out slow, and build up over a period of a week or so. The goal is to get some relief.   No short-term misery for long-term gain. Slow and easy does it.

So What's Wrong With Me?

Well, medically speaking, I have two forms of cancer. One is
fairly benign and takes years to die from. It's called chronic
lymphocytic leukemia. Symptoms are an exceedingly high
white blood count that just keeps going up and up and up.
It took the doctors 59 years to label this disease. The other
cancer I have is ocular metastatic melanoma. It starts in the
eye. When it goes metastatic, it goes to the lung, liver, and
brain. The prognosis is less than six months to live, more
like 6 to 8 weeks.

Given that, a mass was found in my lung back in January,
2012. It measured 3/8" cubed. Since I didn't have health
insurance at that time, I followed up with a biopsy four years
and nine months later in October of 2016. The mass had
grown to 7/8". I'm not a whiz at math, but by my
calculations the mass was growing at the rate of 1/8" per
year. I figure that I've had this metastatic melanoma for 9
years as of 2019. I had a biopsy in 2016, told there was no
treatment, and sent home to die again. I don't know the
size of the mass or where other cancers may have spread in
my body. I figure if they can't treat it, why put myself
through the mind games of "what if."

I have not had radiation done for one simple reason. The
mass is located very, very close to the edge of the lung and
that portion of the lung is directly behind the left ventricle to
my heart. If they radiate the mass, they damage my ability
to pump blood to my heart. I also could have had radiation
to my left eye and stopped the cancer at the source. I lost
my other eye to ocular melanoma 30 years ago before the
cancer had metastasized. Since radiation would blind me in
my only sighted eye, I decided against that. My odds were
better to win the Powerball than to get ocular melanoma in

both eyes. So why aren't I rich?

Chemo? Well, I would have to have two different, highly toxic chemos to kill off the cancer cells in my body before I could go into a clinical trial to receive immunotherapy. I was a lab rat 30 years ago (part of a clinical study) which did not produce any fruitful results. I did not want to ruin my quality of life. I also was not impressed with a clinical trial being done with only 173 participants for immunotherapy. I was not willing to take the risk of side effects of chemo just to have immunotherapy that was not widely tested and die of organ failure. I have never had chemo, but the feedback from friends who did have it said their quality of life drastically changed, or it put them down for the count.

Moving forward, from October of 2017 through November of 2018 I had major problems with my equilibrium. I gave up driving because I didn't want to hurt anyone if I had an accident. I literally bounced off walls. I fainted due to hypoglycemia, so they said. I dieted for months and watched my sugar counts. My energy levels were nonexistent. The nausea was really kicking up. I was living off Zofran and sometimes had to step it up to Phenergan. I started sleeping 16 hours a day. When my sister and husband came to visit, I was a pitiful sight. I had not lost any weight over the years so that was good. However, I couldn't stand the smell of food. I laid on the couch to watch TV with my sister. That was our "we time." I was a barrel of laughs. When she and her husband left at the end of October, they didn't think I'd live through Christmas. Surprise.

But my sister encouraged me to get in touch with my very knowledgeable pharmacist friend who knows all about drugs, supplements (I know, a dirty word) and told her I was failing; it was over. I can hear her now 1,000 miles away. "Not on my watch." So she told me things which I will tell you about in the next chapter.

But before we go there, I will tell you that I followed her instructions to the T. Within 4 weeks, I could stand the smell of food cooking. My nausea was gone. I was able to not only be awake 16 hours a day, but I went back to working from home part-time. My sister is very relieved when she talks with me because she's not getting just yes and no answers. I take her calls when she calls. My energy is not back as far as going shopping, eating out, or entertaining at home. Maybe I'll feel like doing that again someday; maybe I won't. However, I feel like I have quality of life because I can eat, sleep, work, read, or watch TV, all without a tremendous amount of energy being expended or spending my time talking to the porcelain Gods. I actually stay awake and remember what I did during the day and what I watched on TV.

What Are Your Options?

I am going to be brutally honest with you. I don't care how much you like your doctor and his pedigree. S/he will not support your desire to be on supplements. The doctor knows there are thousands of supplements on the market. S/he figures that just because it worked for somebody, that's great, but not his patient. He wants to control every single factor in your treatment.

So if you want to abuse yourself, here's one question to ask your doctor. What are the clinical trial results for extending my life and having quality of life with your advised treatment program? I want to see it in writing.   I can guarantee that you will never see such proof, and he will be highly offended and might even refuse to treat you if you insist on taking supplements.

So what do you do? My advice is to do what you think is right for you. You can allow your physician to play God and totally control your quality of health and life expectancy, or you can weigh all your options, do your own legwork as you're doing now, and decide what you want. Whose life is it anyway?

It is rare for any clinical trial of chemotherapy drugs to extend life let alone give you quality of life. You have trillions of cells. How does chemo or radiation affect the trillions of cells to make sure you're cancer free? MRI's will show masses. PET scans will show hotspots, and some of those hotspots will be false negatives. So back to the question: How do you know when you're cancer free? You don't. You must have a vigilant plan of attack for preventing cancer, and if you have cancer, a plan to keep it at bay. Is that possible?

The melanoma seems, from all CAT scan appearances, to be located in one spot in a single mass in my lung. My understanding, from the doctor who diagnosed me, was that melanoma travels along the optic nerve to the brain, lung, liver and goes everywhere. It does not form masses. Oops. Could there be something else going on? President Carter has metastatic melanoma. From what I can see, his skin reflects there is some sort of problem. I can only assume I'm seeing the results of melanoma. My body has some brown moles here and there, but none are pitch black like the multitudinous ones my mom had with cancer. Obviously my body is treating these cancers differently.

Let's talk about how the medical community responds to treating cancer: Chemo, radiation, surgery. The protocols for some cancers are so aggressive with someone who is just starting to approach stage I cancer, that it's like taking a baseball bat to your countertop to kill an ant, IMHO. My cousin has prostate cancer, not yet at Stage I, however that's defined these days. He has received 37 radiation treatments to his prostate followed by 10 days of rest and then a radiation seed implant put in. Then he takes estrogen shots and 6 other medications.

Back in the day, they used to "watch" cancers like this. So I am SMH (shaking my head) at the baseball bat approach. The health issues it has caused my cousin make it so he can't leave the house. Do you think he will seriously consider chemotherapy just based on what the radiation did to him? He doesn't know. I wouldn't dare advise what anyone should do about treatment. In a way, I feel fortunate that there is no treatment within acceptable risk limits. I might try the immunotherapy, but then again, there are only results for 173 patients and none extended life.

In my humble opinion, some microbiologists might have issues with designing chemotherapy treatments or medications with horrendous side effects. I'm thinking microbiologists, a/k/a scientists, may be going more toward the health and wellness industry because there's some really effective products out there. Doesn't it make sense that these scientists might be able to use their knowledge to create an end product that does not make someone sick? With supplements you don't have to worry about side effects. While there is no guarantee of a cure, an excellent supplement may enable your body to heal itself, which is what your body was designed to do in the first place. With trillions of cells, you need to be realistic, but you may recover some quality of life. However, you will never be cured with supplements or modern medicine.

Bottom line, if you don't like supplements or you want a truckload of documentation offloaded at your doctor's office for his seal of approval, you just wasted five bucks. I am not here to persuade you or convince you to do anything. I'm just telling you what I've done to survive and thrive for 9 years with a deadly cancer that kills in weeks. You can have more quality of life. You just need to do something consistently every single day for your health.

Do I Diet?

Such an ugly word, "diet." However, the ugliest words in the English language are cancer diet. A cancer diet is simple: Spit out anything that tastes good. I would suggest you try that for the first 30 days, like eating raw veggies. But if that idea makes you gag, read on for other options. I eat exactly what I want to.

I decided to not let more than 3 hours go between meals or a healthy snack to keep my blood sugar in balance. *In The Zone* is a great book that gives examples of how everyone should eat. While I can't get excited about their suggestions, I do make myself eat something every three hours. You do not want to starve your body for food as the starvation response sets in in about five hours. Starving yourself only gets the cancer to become aggressive, like poking at a bear.

Basically, each snack, a meal if you can eat that much, should consist of a carbohydrate, protein, and fat. My favorite snack is crackers and cheese. I'm not talking the prepackaged cheese and crackers, but individual crackers from a box and cheese. Preservatives work great when it comes to food, but does nothing for the human body. I have a snack mid-morning, mid-afternoon, and one before I go to bed in addition to three meals. I feel like I'm just shoveling it in all the time. Now that I've gotten to feeling better, I have become aware of how my previous loading up on ice cream, cookies, and homemade breads didn't make me feel as good as I wanted to. My energy levels plummeted. My stomach bothered me. My breathing was labored. So lesson learned. I now can eat what I want and feel so-so to yucky, or I can eat a fairly good diet with regular meals, healthy snacks, and feel decent to good. That's your choice too.

What's Happening in the Body?

It's a widely held belief by those in the health and wellness industry that a junk food diet, a/k/a eating what you like, complex carbs, makes your body acidic. If you've ever seen a green swimming pool, that means that the water has a low pH; it's acidic water. Looks nasty, doesn't it? I imagine that going on inside my body to calm my taste buds from desiring lots of junk food.   I still eat some in moderation, but drink a lot of good water with it.

You may not feel the effects of a low pH, but it's working away in your body. Then you throw in free radicals on top of a low pH. Wonder why you don't feel good? Remember what the green pool water looks like.

What's ideal is to have your body in an alkaline state. I've heard that cancer does not survive in an alkaline state. True or not, it makes sense to me. I just hope the cancer is "going dark." I feel better, so if it's the placebo effect, yeah, team. I doubt it.

FIRST SUGGESTION

So how do you get to that alkaline state without dieting and giving up everything you love to eat? There are a number of things out there, but having a friend who does all the heavy lifting in research for me, her recommendation was pH-FX by Basic Reset. Keep reading before I give you a link. I eat acidic foods in moderation. I just drink pH-FX in with my drinking water (filtered only, please) with my snack and meals. I know I'm cheating, but I think of it as raising my pH as I eat.

pH-FX ($30 plus shipping) is added to filtered water in a PBA free container made by Nalgene. You'll have to Google that to find out where to get one; about $10. The manufacturer of pH-FX recommends a dropper full mixed with 32 ounces of filtered water. I tried half a dropper, and I felt like something the dog should have left in the yard. My pH must have been very low. I had a reaction that lasted three days. I threw the stuff away. Remember, I am very sensitive to medications so I guess I'm sensitive to everything else on the planet except chocolate.

When I could stand suffering no more with extreme nausea, my friend said use baking soda. Well, that was boring a hole in my stomach. So I went back to the pH-FX BUT I used and still use _one or two drops_, _not droppers_, in 32 ounces of water. I am now at full strength with a full dropper. See how that works?

Here's how you know if your pH is up, down, or in between. pH test strips are available at drug stores, Amazon, Walmart. A perfect pH balance is 7.2. Test yourself first. Then keep testing every other day or so to monitor for a pH increase or decrease. If my pH has decreased from the previous test, I drink more pH water. When my pH registers at 8.5 or above, I continue with the same strength and amount of water I was drinking to that point. I'm still not consuming as much pH water as I should be, but my equilibrium and weakness issues are 90% gone.

The manufacturer of this product recommends drinking half your body weight in pH water every day. Remember what I said? Build up slowly to that strength and the amount of pH water you drink. You have no one to blame but yourself if you don't feel good.

Testing your urine and saliva. Drink this water with meals, snacks, especially when eating acidic foods, such as fruit, but it basically includes everything you eat except a blade of grass.

Directions:
1. Shake pH-FX bottle (the source) every time before mixing up a new batch of pH water.
2. Add filtered water.
3. Use PBA free bottle.
The website link is http:basicreset.com. I make no money off any sale of this product, nor do I have any ownership interest in the company. The cost is $30 plus shipping and tax. It has lasted me a couple of months.

SECOND SUGGESTION

Let's talk about water intake. It is a necessity to keep a clean colon, period. Fecal matter is toxic. It drains my energy levels tremendously if I don't throughput what I eat. I try to make sure to get at least half my body weight in water intake every day. Constipation is a terrible thing to live with. I get pain, nausea, as well as other nasty things happen.   You can't get your body to an alkaline state when you're full of it. So water, water, water. Also, I can easily tell myself that every single symptom, including a hangnail, is a sign the cancer is spreading. I doubt that that's true, LOL, but since I've been diagnosed with cancer, I have a tendency to think the worst when a new ache or pain or symptom arises.

THIRD SUGGESTION

I use oxygen 24/7. I find it boosts my energy levels for the hours I'm up and makes me steadier on my feet, like it reduces the unsteadiness and dizziness in late-stage cancer. It helps me sleep better. I've also heard that it's good to oxygenate your cells. I don't know the science, but it works for me. When you get admitted to Hospice, you can have anything you want, so just ask. I'll skip tranquilizers any day for oxygen.

A couple things I was never told when I started using oxygen is maintenance of the equipment. Oversight. ☐

First, use distilled water in the humidifier bottle.

Two, once a week take the humidifier bottle out of the concentrator, empty the water out and dry the bottle. Then refill it with distilled water to the fill mark and start your engines.

Three, change your tubing and nasal canula out once a month. There's no way to clean these things.   I can only imagine the bacteria buildup of something you insert in your nose and wear every day. Ewwww.

Four, water trap. This little contraption is attached to the oxygen tubing as the last connection before your nasal cannula tubing. To put it in the middle between two 25-foot cords will cause problems such as, I felt like I was being waterboarded with excess water bubbling in my nostrils and choking me. It sounded like someone was making popcorn in my nose. Apparently this doesn't bother some people, but it wakes me up out of sound sleep. I buy them off eBay, brand name, Salter Labs. When you see water accumulating in the trap itself, empty it, or just do it every eight hours.

Five, I use the small adult canula. I do not have a big nose.
If I use an adult canula, especially being a side sleeper, it
flares out my nostrils, or one side pops out and oxygen only
goes in my nose on one side, and I feel very uncomfortable.

How do you get the kinks and coils out of the oxygen hose?
You can upgrade from plastic tubing to vinyl which doesn't
kink as bad. The second idea, I found on the internet, tried
it, and it works. I get a bag that zips up, like a pillow case
cover or lingerie bag, and put the hose in the bag. I put the
bag in the dryer with several towels (I use bath towels) and
I set the dryer on medium heat for 15 minutes. When I take
the bag out of the dryer, I immediately take the hose out
and run my fingers over it to smooth it out while extending it
so the hose will lay flat. It works. If you don't leave it in
there long enough, it doesn't turn out well. If you have a
really hot dryer, you can burn your fingers and perhaps melt
the tubing, so be careful.

What Else Am I Doing?

Let's start out with a general explanation before we get to the details. One, I learned from my resources that free radical damage causes most diseases: Cancer, Alzheimer's, senility, arthritis, diabetes, heart disease and more. When you have cancer treatments, you are getting exposed to free radicals whether the source is chemo or radiation. Think of free radical damage as oxidative stress, like rust on a radiator. Eventually the rust particles all pile up in one place and spread out, kind of like a metastasis. Now you need a new radiator. If you did something about the first little rust spot, you would not have had such a big repair bill. If cancer could be detected and treated before it turned into a mass, or we could do something that was effective to help address free radical damage, would we be sick?

From what I've been told, the supplement I take neutralizes 1,000,000,000 free radicals a second and kicks on your survival genes. Plus each pill lasts in your system for 13 days. So think about it. The free radicals are neutralized and, therefore, do not need to be processed by your liver to get them out of your body. This is very good. If you've had chemo, your liver is highly toxic so you don't need to be adding more toxic matter to your liver.

Now, if you're saying to yourself, if this stuff is so good why won't my doctor recommend it, ask him or her. Ask him to prove that it <u>won't</u> work. Trying to prove a negative is difficult and expect acting out by your doctor. They don't like being questioned. At this point, you have a decision to make. Tell your doctor or not. I doubt if your doctor can neutralize free radicals (that cause disease) at 1,000,000 a second; 60,000,000 in a minute; 360,000,000 in an hour or give you something nontoxic that kicks on your survival genes. Hmn.

With cancer, you want to neutralize the free radical damage, the rust, going on inside your body. After hours and hours of research, my friend recommended I take **Protandim Blue Bottle**. I take two pills a day, seven hours apart, with meals. One bottle contains 30 pills, costs $50 and lasts one month (30 pills). This product has been clinically studied by 29 universities and extensively peer reviewed. I bought the product and tried it for 90 days back in 2012. I'm still taking it.

Go online and go to www.LifeVantage.com.   You'll have to create an account. No worries. No one will bug you with calls. You may be able to buy it on Amazon, but you have no idea how the product has been stored or if there's been a recall on the product for some reason. It is tested and withstands GMP, good manufacturing principles.

Did you realize your body makes its own anti-oxidants? If you're eating a fairly good diet, why would I need to supplement with anti-oxidants? To me, it's a waste of money to take a number of supplements when one pill will do the job very effectively. If you insist, don't take them all at one sitting. Take them an hour apart because you don't know how they will interact. I have a friend who throws them all in one big slushy. She has not felt well for the past two years. She stopped the Protandim since "it wasn't doing anything," I suggested she try an hour of separation between all her vast number of supplements. She suggested that I mind my own business. All I take for my two cancers are Protandim and pH-FX. That is it.

WARNING: Like anything you put in your body, whether food, medications, or supplements, you *could have* a reaction. Reactions are extremely rare, but there's always somebody who will get a reaction and go ballistic on the person who suggested it and the company. I'm not a blamer. I'm cautious. Just remember how sensitive I said I

am to everything ingested. So I started by taking a portion
of the Protandim pill, like a fourth of one the first day. Then
I titrated up over a week's time to a whole pill. Many, many
people have taken this safely, but **common sense must
prevail**. I would stop taking all other supplements to make
sure there are no interactions. I've never taken any other
supplements or vitamins, and I'm 9 years out with a very
deadly cancer and leukemia.

While we're on the topic of taking multiple supplements, I
want to pass on a story that you need to hear. If you're
taking different supplements together, it's like drinking a
hairy buffalo, you know, all the booze left at the end of the
party combined in one container and you drink it. No. You
don't know how supplements will interact. If you insist,
please take your supplement one hour away from any other
supplement and/or medication.   Drink some pH water with it
for optimal results.

(I know there are arguments out there and someone may
want to arm wrestle me about T-bars. Don't bother. The
supplement cannot be tested that way, but oxidative stress
load levels are phenomenally reduced after 30 days. This
was a peer reviewed study by PubMed.)

Technically, your body produces all the antioxidants it needs
all by itself. I've read that taking more antioxidants in pill
form are useless. What you're trying to do is take care of
the present free radical damage you have in your body and
neutralize it as well as fight new free radical damage.
Protandim neutralizes 1,000,000 free radicals a second. Yes,
you read that right, per second. The pill will last up to 13
days in your body, which is why I said go slow when you
start.

But consider this. If you've taken 13 pills, one a day over 2
weeks, you have 13,000,000 free radicals being neutralized

per second at the end of two weeks. You do the math because my old calculator blew up on that number. Now try two pills a day and in two weeks you'll have 26,000,000 free radicals a second being neutralized. It only makes sense to me that you'll feel better once you're neutralizing free radical damage to your body. If you are going the chemo and radiation route because you feel that is your best option, just know that these treatments are creating massive free radical damage. My thinking is, and it's only my opinion, that once the radiation blast is over and/or the chemo treatment is over, why couldn't a person take Protandim? After 24 hours, the chemo has done all it's going to do which is kill off cells, good or bad, because it can't distinguish between the two.

Your oncologist could take exception to everything I've said here. As a matter of fact, I don't know of one who wouldn't. It's like trying to get Democrats and Republicans to agree. Again, it's your choice to take a leap of faith into the great unknown. I lost my lifelong best friend because she believed chemo had been keeping her alive. She took another supplement when Protandim was not available. It was very, very expensive, **but** her counts greatly improved. The oncologist said her success was due to the chemo treatment she received six months before, and it had finally worked. LOL. He was taking all the credit for what a supplement did. She told him about the supplement, and he told her to get off the supplement immediately if she wanted more chemo. Nice emotional blackmail. Her story gets much more sordid after this experience. After quitting the supplement, she became deathly ill before passing six months later.

If you would like to go on YouTube, put in Dr. Marvin Protandim in the search box. He has several presentations out there. Now, be prepared. He is older, in his 80s, and speaks like Carlton, the Doorman, bless his heart. He is very knowledgeable on Protandim and has lots of videos out there for your entertainment and scientific pleasure.

So you make the call on what you want to do. The big bucks are in oncology and radiation. If I didn't get so sick off a Tylenol, I might have considered chemo as an option. I have lived far past my expiration date.

One last thing. What's so great about <u>neutralizing</u> free radicals is that there is no toxic cleansing going on in your liver or your blood. Nasty free radicals are neutralized. Since I'm not scientifically savvy on how Protandim works, I would think that while it neutralizes free radicals, it might neutralize free radicals in the liver, brain or anywhere else. Why not?

In conclusion, I don't think it's an accident that my metastatic melanoma has not advanced rapidly over the last 9 years. The epicenter of the cancer is in my only remaining sighted eye. That's why I started taking Protandim, because I didn't want to go blind. I still see well, wear a contact lens and have for 56 years.

SUGGESTION FOR SKIN CARE DURING RADIATION TREATMENTS

This is a bonus tip for those of you undergoing radiation, for your delicate skin. Radiation is no different from laying in the sun day after day with a UV 10 and no sun screen. You will burn, and it will hurt. A friend of mine used a lotion with aloe in it called Emprizone which is made by Mannatech out of Dallas, Texas, http:mannatech.com. After 35 or so radiation treatments, they asked her to do another 10 treatments to make sure they got it all. She was sore from the radiation, but controlled the burn. Another friend did nothing to protect her breast and was left with a shriveled up mess.   Naturally you don't want a heavy duty cream on your breast or testicles or whatever is being radiated because that might act like putting on baby oil instead of sun screen. Emprizone washes off easily so you could do that right before your treatment and put it right back on afterward.

SUGGESTIONS AFTER CHEMO OR RADIATION

If you felt uneasy about using any supplement during treatment, use it now that you're done with treatment. I feel for those of you who have become incontinent because of treatment, but without anything in your system to protect you, it will happen. It's time now to get the free radical damage taken care of in your body. Chemo kills good cells as well as cancer cells. Therefore, there's a lot of mopping up to do. A health professional told me years ago that after three treatments, your liver puts up a figurative stop sign. It can't handle anymore toxicity. What happens? The toxic stuff backs up into your blood. Naturally you're going to feel like something hanging off the dog's butt that you wish was in the yard. However, attack it now with the Protandim and the pH water. You've got nothing to lose, IMHO. I've seen it work for others. Congrats if you had the option and the guts to take chemo. It was not an option for me, but bless others who can.

So Now What?

What has kept me sane and positive during those 16 months of equilibrium issues and pass outs, nausea, blah, blah, is, I keep as normal a routine as possible. I was obviously housebound, and I remain so to this day by choice. If you've ever lived in the Bible Belt, you'd understand. I felt like if I could work, then I could tolerate my existence without a lot of crying and whining. So let's talk about a couple of things.

Self-limiting beliefs will set you on a course to be a self-fulfilling prophecy. If the doctor says you have six months to live and you believe him, then you will only have six months or less to live. What's happened in this scenario is the doctor has taken away all your hope. I chose not to believe the jackass the first time I had melanoma. He didn't have any evidence of that statement because he did no testing, just looked in my eye. He lined my parents up against the wall of the exam room, and said, she has 6 to 8 weeks to live so get her affairs in order.

Needless to say, my dad made sure I got another opinion from the top doctor in the country. No doctor will mess with his kid. The second time I got cancer, I went about living my life and moved 1,800 miles across the country to live in a place with a lower cost of living. My belief was and still is, the doctor is not in control of my body or my mindset. However, I am in control with a lot of help from the good Lord. I have the power to decide if the balance of my days, however many or few days there are, will be happy days, well days if I can get them with supplements, or sick days from treatment.

So let's talk about the initial reaction you get when you get the diagnosis. Fear. I can't think of one person who said, oh, yeah, I look forward to dying of cancer. Nope. Never. My lifelong best friend told me, it's not dying that's hard, it's the process.

So now that you are checking out your options for quality of life, take action to improve your health. When I started to see some progress, like I didn't pass out if I stood up fast, then my fear levels subsided. My greatest fear stemmed from the pass outs and potential blindness. Once I was diagnosed with chronic lymphocytic leukemia, I was immediately put in the Hospice program. I've been at home leading my life thanks to the nurses, personal assistant, chaplain, social worker, LPN and medical director. They are phenomenal people who are ever so helpful and supportive. They're amazed at what they're seeing here which leads me to my next topic.

Faith. You may say, I don't believe in God or Jesus for whatever reason. I'll bet when you start having symptoms of decline, you will become a believer. You'll be crying out, oh, God, help me. Say what you want, but life gets a whole lot easier when you have faith.   God's available 24/7 and is always ready, willing, and able to help you if you give him more than lip service.

I'd rather believe that God, Jesus, and the Holy Spirit exist than take the chance that they don't. Since my diagnoses, I regularly need my fears to be calmed. I don't need stress and neither do you. Medications make things worse for me because they make me sick. I'm doing this alone with no one within 1,400 miles. Therefore, fear is very real for me. I want to be able to take care of myself, cook, do laundry, work, and take care of my home until my last breath and die peacefully in my sleep. Isn't that what we all want? It just doesn't happen that way for everybody.   So I pray a lot. I certainly have the time.

I finally feel like my heart is right with God. Now if I could just keep on praying for political leaders to be able to come together and agree on what's good for this country. Sometimes I get so angry, negative, and depressed. I have no control over the USA let alone any individual politician. I have no control over cancer. I have to let things go. Control is highly overrated. We are not God. We cannot force a solution to all or even most of life's problems whether in our relationships, finances, home, or the political environment in the USA or anywhere else in the world. God gave us free will, so let's use our free will as an asset instead of a liability. Get your relationships right that have soured with others, or at the very least, forgive yourself for what you think you've done wrong. Forgive yourself for your flaws, and thank God for every day above ground.

One little daily inspirational message book I have used since 2010 might help you. It's called *Jesus Calling* by Sarah Young. 25 million copies have been sold. One message a day, 365 days, and it's rarely more than a page long and has big print. There are a couple Bible verses (not chapters) after the message. Be sure to read the introduction to the book or you'll be scratching your head. It helps me tremendously.

As far as church goes, I attend Dr. Stanley's church online. He gets the message across in 25 minutes and talks from his heart. If he's not your speed, go find someone else to listen to. Just do something to feed your soul.

So that's it for my big protocol for what I'm doing to get quality of life. Getting into the latter stages of cancer, my body tells me what I'm going to do, not the other way around. I sleep when I'm tired. I work, cook, do laundry when I'm not tired.   No guilt, no stress.

CAREGIVERS

Who do you look to as a caregiver?

This is a question that has haunted me for a long time. I have one relative left so Hospice has been doing the initial caregiving since I'm still ambulatory and have quality of life. However, even though I'm feeling very alone and frightened of the process, I know that allowing a new person into my life is the most dangerous thing I could do right now. Due to my lifelong career in court reporting, I have seen horror stories happen when you allow someone new into your life when you are so vulnerable. I don't want to end up being thrown out of my house, car taken, checking account emptied, et cetera, all because I trusted the wrong person in end times.   Most days I don't have a lot of spare energy to care. While watching the TV 24/7 is boring, it's so much safer than a stranger in the house. Yes, they may appear very caring. However, back before all the cancer hit, I was royally taken advantage of by men and women so I would not trust my judgment in that regard anymore. If this is your situation, I do hope there is a relative you can trust to help you out.

When do you ask a caregiver to step in?

Next to the previous question, this is the next hardest question to answer. My caregivers would have to travel 1400 miles to get to me. How long would they have to stay? I'm uprooting them from their lives while they are with me. When do I ask?   The answer is: Have the decision made by your caregiver before the situation happens. That way, you don't feel like a burden.

Also, if the caregiver decides to be there for you, you have fulfilled your responsibility of allowing them to be there. Read that again. You do have a responsibility with regards to your final days, weeks, months, of not shutting out the people who love you and who want to be there for you. That can be so hurtful when you exclude them from your life. As you can see, having a frank talk before the caregiver needs to step in is essential to take the stress off you.

Special Information for Caregivers:

1. When a cancer patient gets toward their end days, when their quality of life is minimal, this is when you need to be strong emotionally so you can put on your most loving face and give your most encouraging support. While you don't want to totally curb the patient's independence, you don't want them to hurt themselves either. A fall during this time may occur whether the patient has balance issues or not as they are very weak. A fall could require admittance into a nursing home if a bone is broken as you might not be able to handle the lifting required to get the patient in and out of bed for bathroom or porta-potty use. Broken bones do not heal very quickly, if at all, with cancer.

2.   How to get the patient to consider Hospice care at home.   This may be easier than you think. Once the fatigue, nausea, and/or total body weakness starts, the patient does not want to go out. Therefore, you approach the patient from the point of view that, you will never have to go to the doctor's office or ER again. Everything can be taken care of at home. That worked on my mom. Boom. Hospice was on scene shortly.

If this approach doesn't work, then your loved one has not accepted the reality of their situation. Calling on a minister, social worker (all available through Hospice) may help the patient with their decision. My best friend fought cancer for 13 years and still wanted more chemo as she thought it would save her life. No one was going to change her mind. Therefore, be sure you go with your cancer patient to the doctor's office for a visit when the patient's health begins to decline. Introduce yourself at the appointment. Ask to see the doctor privately without the patient present. Then out of earshot of the cancer patient, tell the doctor what's going on and ask if s/he will note on the chart to order Hospice in at the family's request. Be sure it's on the chart notes or patient file so it can be ordered from those notes. That way if the doctor is on a cruise to the Orient, you don't have to wait for him/her to get back.

3.   Points to consider in caregiving:
       a. If my loved one is sleeping, should I let him/her know I'm there and ask if they want to go to the bathroom, if they want to eat? Let sleeping dogs lie. I say this because sleep can be evasive to a cancer patient. Being in bed 24/7 and dealing with symptoms makes a cancer patient very restless. The body isn't used to it. The body is starting to shut down. In my mom's final days, I just let her sleep.

       b.   Hospice gives the best advice on when and how to medicate. You don't want to ever have your loved one suffer with breakthrough pain more than once. That is a heart-wrenching experience you will never forget.   So do you have to wake them up to give them their meds? Not if you have liquid medication you can administer for pain and anxiety. You just put in a <u>little bit</u> under the tongue where it is absorbed into the bloodstream.

4. When you have to change the sheets or whatever they're wearing to help with incontinence, it's decision time. If you are not able to move them by yourself, then you may need some cooperation from the patient. If you have help, problem solved. With high pain levels, this is difficult on you emotionally, but your logic tells you it has to be done. So pre-medicate for pain in order to alleviate the patient's discomfort. Again, ask Hospice for advice.

5. When the patient is sleeping, you can be with them.
Hold their hand gently. Talk to them very softly, whether
you think they can hear you or not. It's comforting to the
patient. But don't ask questions like, are you in pain.
Hospice should have already advised you as to how much
pain meds you can give and when. You don't need to ask
about giving meds unless the patient has previously stated
they don't want meds except on request.

6. I don't know about other cancer patients, but the smell of
food cooking can be nauseating. So the best time to cook
something is when the patient is sleeping soundly. If you
want fish, I advise you cook it elsewhere and bring it home.
That smell is offensive to some people and the smell can last
for days.

7. Choose a funeral home. When your loved one has
passed, you definitely <u>call Hospice first</u> (when the patient's at
home) so the RN can pronounce the patient and notifies the
doctor who will be filling out a death certificate when
presented with it by the funeral home. Then, and only then,
<u>Hospice calls the funeral home</u>. Please say all your
goodbyes before you call Hospice. Do not hold the funeral
home up from taking your loved one because your family is
coming in from all over the area to say goodbye just so you
can avoid the cost of a private visitation at the funeral home.
Some families do this in order to avoid paying for
embalming, which is not required in cremation. However, to
see a body at the funeral home, states require embalming in
order to prevent the spread of disease. It's for your
protection.

8. Join a bereavement support group. Hospice can
recommend one. It's good to grieve at or around the time of
your loss. When my husband passed, I didn't grieve for 18
months because I was so busy trying to just survive. Then it
hit like a freight train. I was in bed for six months and lost

25 pounds. Delayed grief syndrome is a very serious condition.

9. **TAKE CARE OF YOURSELF AS A CAREGIVER!!!**

You need to follow the same protocol as the patient. If your family has a history of Alzheimer's, cancer, diabetes, heart disease, et cetera, you can change your history. Medications mask symptoms; an excellent supplement can enable your body to heal itself when it is taken on a preventative basis. Go to page 11 for my two suggestions to stay healthy and strong. You won't regret it. Plus, you'll need a strong body to help you through a demanding time of your life.

If you have to be "on" 24/7 for healthcare, ask the family to kick in for a sitter or home healthcare person to take over during the hours you need to sleep. If you're having problems sleeping, ask your doctor for something to help you sleep. While this is not an easy task you've decided to undertake, I promise you it will be the most rewarding thing you will ever do. You can look back and realize that no matter what issues you may have had previously in your life with the patient, you came through for them when they needed you most. All is forgiven.

At this point in your process of doing the best you can for yourself and coordinate the best decisions for medical care, you have to do what is right for you. Do your research. Do the homework that's required to make an intelligent decision that is not based on just what your oncologist tells you. If I had relied on that, I don't know if I'd be here to tell you how things are turning out for me. It's a very personal decision that only you can make. I have no skin in the game, no dollars invested, no sales pitch for you to listen to ad nauseum. This is about your desire to live as healthy a life as possible until you take your last breath. Whose life is it anyway?

Now, what worked for me may not work for you especially if the cancer is in your bone marrow. Like I said, I also have chronic lymphocytic leukemia. That's in the bone marrow. I could take the really pricey supplement or just keep on doing with what I've been doing. Seeing how the last 8 out of the 10 years were very good to me and I only discovered the pH water three months ago, I'm doing pretty good.

Everybody measures quality of life differently. As far as I'm concerned and with how far I slid until I started using the pH water, I feel like I received a miracle. I can eat, eliminate, sleep, sit up, watch TV, talk with people and all with no ill effects. I can withstand strong cooking odors without gagging. Do I go dancing, shopping and out to eat? No. One, because I don't have the energy I would like to have to do that. Two, I don't need to be exposed to all the germs out there because with any form of leukemia, germ exposure needs to be limited. Three, I now live in the Bible Belt and don't know a soul. All men have the same name, I'm married. I didn't proposition you, dummy. I just asked your name so I could say thank you for getting that box off the top shelf at the grocery. Duh.

All kidding aside, I'm happy to be alive. I'm grateful for every day, and hope there will be more days, particularly good days, maybe some great days. Having cancer or any other dreaded disease gives you a whole new outlook on life. Most people have a paradigm shift from the way they used to think. Now, family and relationships are a top priority. I'm grateful I'm still able to work. I don't work a lot, but I work enough to pay my bills. That feeling of independence where you're shouting, don't put dirt on my grave just yet, is more than a hit song. It rings true for those of us who are surviving. Now let's see if we can thrive.

EPILOGUE

I wish I had the time and energy to sit down with everyone who gets this book who reads it, and takes it to heart. I had to charge $5.50 for it to get onto Amazon because otherwise I would have had to get a web site, blog, search engine position, a blog, blah, blah. If you like what you read, pass it along to others.   If I gave it away for free, someone would only copy it and charge money for it. Therefore, you might as well get the true story from the source. I don't know of anyone diagnosed with ocular metastatic melanoma and chronic lymphocytic leukemia simultaneously.

When you get right down to it, the cost of the two items that have helped me is pretty nominal. You have a choice to come up with excuses, or come up with the money. One lady who suffered vicious migraines didn't have the money. Well, I can't help you with that. All I know is, I used to have migraines, took a supplement, and within six months I didn't have migraines ever again. You figure it out because the decision is square on your shoulders.

Remember what I said. We live on a toxic planet. Sometimes you see family members getting a specific cancer that mom or dad had. Guess what? They were all exposed to the same toxins while growing up together. You don't know what that was, but it happened. You suffered from free radical damage and were never able to do anything about it. Now you can.

Whatever your decision, I wish you the very best.

www.ingramcontent.com/pod-product-compliance
Lightning Source LLC
Chambersburg PA
CBHW051427250726
48655CB00003B/1286